Homemade

A Complete Beginner's Guide to

Natural DIY Shampoos you can

Make Today

Jane Aniston

<u>Introduction</u>

Thank you for choosing to download this book; *"Homemade Shampoo - A Complete Beginner's Guide to Natural DIY Shampoos You Can Make Today"*.

Here you'll find all the information you need in order to start making your own natural, chemical-free shampoos at home today. The vast majority of the ingredients used to make these shampoos are cheap and easily available, and the process of making the shampoos couldn't be simpler!

In this book, we'll cover the differences between homemade shampoos and store-bought shampoos and show you why you really should ditch expensive, toxic, store-bought shampoos and start making your own natural, healthy, chemical-free shampoos at home.

This book also includes 34 natural shampoo recipes. Each recipe will list the ingredients required to make the shampoo and then guide you through the process of exactly what you'll need to do, with simple, easy to follow, step by step instructions, meaning you'll be making your own shampoos in no time at all!

Once you see how clean and healthy natural homemade shampoos can keep your hair, you'll never want to go back to harmful store-bought shampoos which can be toxic not only to your hair and your body but also the environment.

Thank you again for downloading this book. I hope you enjoy it!

Jane Aniston

responsibility or blame be held against the publisher for any reparation, damages, or monetary loss due to the information herein, either directly or indirectly.

Respective authors own all copyrights not held by the publisher.

The information herein is offered for informational purposes solely, and is universal as so. The presentation of the information is without contract or any type of guarantee assurance.

The trademarks that are used are without any consent, and the publication of the trademark is without permission or backing by the trademark owner. All trademarks and brands within this book are for clarifying purposes only and are the owned by the owners themselves, not affiliated with this document.

Table of contents

3. Peppermint and Rosemary Shampoo

4. Lavender and Bergamot Milky Mix

5. Avocado Aloe Surprise

6. A Little Bit of Sunshine

7. Surprisingly Good Apple & Garlic Shampoo

8. Shining Shimmering Splendid Shampoo

9. Lovely Lemony Egg Shampoo

10. Miraculous Apple Cider Shampoo

11. Awesome Aromatherapy Shampoo

12. Chamomile and Apricot Shampoo

13. Shiny Strawberry Shampoo

14. Anti-Damage Shampoo

15. Merry Minty Rosemary

Chapter 5: Homemade Shampoos for Dry Hair

34. Dry Baking Soda and Oatmeal Shampoo

Conclusion

A message from the author, Jane Aniston

Chapter 1

Why You Should Stop Using Store-bought Shampoos and Start Making Your Own Natural Shampoos at Home!

There are hundreds of shampoos on the market and each one of them promises to leave your hair shinier, softer and more beautiful than the rest. Realistically though, these shampoos rarely live up to their lofty promises, and in fact, for a number of reasons that we'll go into in this book, by far the best option is to simply make your own natural shampoos at home.

While the vast majority of us grow up believing that using store-bought shampoos is the only option, it's never too late to understand that there is actually a better alternative. After thoroughly investigating store-bought shampoos, I highly recommend you give making your own toxin-free, natural homemade shampoos a try, as these products are far better for your hair, your health, and the environment.

You're probably wondering why you should spend the extra time and energy to make your own shampoos when you can easily grab a bottle off the shelf in your local supermarket? Well, here's a rundown of facts that will help you understand why homemade shampoos are most definitely better than the store-bought variety!

1. **Natural homemade shampoos take fantastic care of your hair.** Contrary to popular belief, it isn't necessary to wash our hair with chemical shampoo every day. The reason for this is that over-shampooing strips the hair of it's natural oils, and due to their harshness, this is particularly true of store-bought shampoos. However, when you begin using homemade shampoos you'll notice that your hair will look healthier and that the right amount of protective natural oils will remain intact.

2. **You can make natural homemade shampoos in small amounts and keep them in non-polluting, reusable containers until you need them.** Most of the shampoos in this book can be stored in the fridge for at least a few days, and up to a couple of weeks, saving you from having to regularly make new batches. Although a regular shampoo container can be used to store your homemade shampoos, the best way of storing them is in glass containers. The reason for this is that glass is inert meaning no chemicals can leach out into your shampoos. As these containers are reusable and made of non-toxic material you'll also have the peace of mind that you're not just doing what's right for your hair, but also what's right for the environment!

3. **Store-bought shampoos are often full of potentially cancer-causing chemicals.** As we are all well aware, cancer is a truly awful disease! Therefore it's important that we do whatever we can in order to reduce the risk of ever suffering from this terrible condition. Cocamide DEA, a chemical found in nearly a hundred types of store-bought shampoos in the USA, has a proven link to the formation of cancerous cells in humans. Most shampoos also contain vast amounts of sulfates and parabens that may poison the scalp and the kidneys, and could also play a part in the onset of allergies. When you're using store-bought shampoos, you're exposing yourself to a vast array of chemical nasties, and in so doing you're putting yourself at risk of potentially

damaging your body's tissues and organs. Other chemicals to beware of include:

- **Formaldehyde.** Yes, that's the same formaldehyde used for embalming the dead! While it may be OK for the dead, it's certainly not something we want to be introducing into our bodies while we're still alive! Formaldehyde can play a part in cancer formation and can reportedly cause our body's organs to stiffen. This in turn may contribute to the onset of organ damage.

- **Sodium Lauryl Sulphate.** This chemical slowly damages the hair by breaking down it's natural protein structure. An additional downside is that it can in some cases lead to lung or eye irritation.

- **Polyoxyethylene, Sodium Chloride, and other Thickening Agents.** These chemical agents are used to help shampoo lather easily. However, they can actually cause your scalp to become dry and itchy as they remove the natural oils which work to keep the hair and scalp healthy.

- **Synthetic Colors.** These chemicals can cause irritation of the scalp and skin.

- **Siloxane, Dimethicone, Silicone and other Hair Sealants.** These ingredients are reported to make the hair shiny, but due to their harsh chemical nature they can actually prevent the scalp from being able to coat hair with it's natural oils. This in turn can lead to dry, frizzy and hard-to-manage hair.

- **Mineral Oil, Petroleum, and Lanolin.** While these products claim to moisturize your hair, they actually have no proven benefits. Like most chemicals in commercially available shampoos, they can strip away the natural oils and moisture from the hair and in extreme cases may even cause the hair to thin or, at worst, fall out!

- **Propylene Glycol or Anti-Freeze Agents.** You may be wondering (as I was when I first found out), "Why on earth would there be anti-freeze in my shampoo!?" Well, quite simply it's used in order to stop the shampoo from freezing while in transport. This is the same anti-freeze that you might use in your car and, needless to say, it`s NOT something that you want to be rubbing into your scalp! Anti-freezing agents may cause allergic reactions as well as skin irritation.

- **Alcohol.** The relatively high amounts of alcohol found in some of the shampoos available on store shelves may dry the hair and make it heavy and brittle.

As you can see, there are a wide range of potentially harmful ingredients in some store-bought shampoos. If we really care about the health of our hair and our bodies, perhaps we should think twice about using them and give alternative options a chance.

4. **Natural homemade shampoos are packed full of natural goodness.** A lot of people are going organic these days when it comes to their diets. While it's important to be concerned about what we eat and drink, it's also important to think about what we are

applying to other parts of our bodies. When we use natural products on our hair, we don't only look good, we can also be sure that we'll feel good, too. Some of the wonderful ingredients that we can use in our natural homemade shampoos include:

- **Apricot.** A natural nourishing agent that's not only good for soothing the skin, it's actually great for the hair too.

- **Avocado.** Avocado contains lots of great natural fats and proteins that can play a big part in helping to keep our hair looking healthy and lustrous.

- **Chamomile.** Chamomile is not only soothing, it also smells great and revitalizes the hair!

- **Honey.** Honey acts as a natural hair softener and gives the hair a beautiful shine.

- **Coconut Milk.** Coconut milk has been used by people for centuries to help keep their hair looking and feeling soft and smooth. You'll notice that a couple of shampoo recipes in this book contain coconut milk; it really is a fantastic ingredient to use in your homemade shampoos!

- **Fenugreek.** A very powerful Indian herb which has anti-fungal and revitalizing properties. This ingredient could be a little difficult to find, but if you decide to take the time to source it you can be sure that it will definitely be worth the effort!

- **Rosemary.** Because of it's great smell and its calming properties, rosemary can help to relax us. For this reason it's used in numerous recipes within this book. Luckily, it's super easy to find in almost any supermarket and it combines well with almost any of the other ingredients.

- **Peppermint.** Peppermint can leave your hair and scalp feeling fresh and cool. It's also said that peppermint can play a part in helping hair grow faster.

- **Mint.** Has similar revitalizing and cooling effects to peppermint.

- **Strawberry.** Strawberries contain natural compounds that are extremely nourishing for both the hair and scalp, so adding a few strawberries to your homemade shampoo a sure way to create a shampoo which will leave your hair lustrous and healthy!

- **Tea Tree Oil.** This amazing, natural antibiotic is a marvel of nature! It leaves the hair with a silky shine and can even act as a natural insect repellent, driving away bugs such as mosquitoes! A truly brilliant ingredient for your homemade shampoos and for your bathroom cabinet if you ever have cuts or blemishes!

- **Arrowroot.** The hair needs protein to grow and Arrowroot will help provide this protein via the scalp. Also said to strengthen the hair.

- **Shikakai.** This Indian ingredient is sure to bring your crowning glory back to life due to it's invigorating qualities.

- **Coconut Oil.** Coconut Oil can help restore our hair's natural health, giving it a fantastic shine and suppling the hair and scalp with natural oils.

- **Ylang-Ylang.** Ylang-Ylang is best used in shampoos for washing hair at night as it is calming and relaxing. It also helps the hair retain natural vitamins, minerals, and oils.

- **Jasmine.** Has similar effects to Ylang-Ylang but is also said to put anyone who smells it in a romantic mood!

- **Rose.** Rose has a wonderful fragrance. and can also have a positive effect on hair growth.

- **Curry spices.** Surprising as it sounds, curry contains protein that the hair can make use of via the scalp.

- **Lavender.** Lavender is calming and leaves hair smelling fresh. Shampoos containing lavender are best used at night as the scent of lavender is known to promote a restful night's sleep.

- **Aloe Vera.** Another of nature's marvels, aloe-vera can restore even the limpest of hair, giving it a fresh, vibrant appearance after just a few washes!

- **Baking Soda**. A versatile ingredient that can be used to make the most basic natural shampoo. (See Chapter 3 for more on this.) After reading this book you'll never look at plain old baking soda in the same way again!

- **Eggs.** Act as a natural moisturizer.

- **Olive oil.** This wonderful, health-promoting favorite of those who enjoy Mediterranean-style meals is also fantastic for adding moisture to your hair and helping to restore it's natural oil balance.

These are just some of the amazing ingredients that you can use to make your own shampoos. As you read through this book you'll see that there are many more ingredients, either around your home or easily available at the local supermarket, that you can use to make incredible, natural shampoos.

5. **Natural homemade shampoos are fragrant without being overpowering.** If you're anything like me you may find the smell

of some store-bought shampoos overpowering! As mentioned earlier, small particles of the harsh chemicals used in commercial shampoos can irritate your hair and scalp, but in addition, they can also play havoc with your nostrils! When you make your own natural shampoos, not only do you avoid dodgy chemicals, you're also able to decide the scent of your shampoo by including your favorite essential oils and fragrance oils. In so doing, you'll be able to make a bespoke shampoo that's tailored to your specific preferences, both in terms of the results it produces as well as the fragrance it emits. You can even make a variety of shampoos with different scents and then select the one which best suits you at the time of washing your hair; an invigorating fragrance to freshen you up while you're taking your morning shower and a calming shampoo to relax you before bed.

6. **Natural homemade shampoos may help you feel better** For all these years, you've been introducing toxic compounds to your body via your scalp on an almost daily basis. While we may not be aware of the effects this is having on us, it's very possible that over the years the chemicals in our shampoos have built up in our systems and played a part in leaving us susceptible to illness. When we start making our own healthy shampoos, we are able to let go of this worrying thought as we know that we're using nothing but natural, health-promoting ingredients to clean our hair and scalp.

7. **Natural homemade shampoos are less expensive than store-bought shampoos, and they're fun to make!** Going the DIY route is favored by many, not only because of the aforementioned benefits, but simply because it's such good fun! Instead of going to the store and spending over the odds for a bottle of mystery-soap, you can spend an enjoyable morning or afternoon making your own natural products. And when you have a little more experience you can experiment by mixing and matching ingredients to find the combinations that are best suited to you, meaning you'll be creating your very own, one-of-a-kind hair care products!

As you've seen, there are so many reasons why you should try making your own homemade shampoos. Homemade shampoos aren't just good for you, they're also great for the environment, giving you the peace of mind that, in a small way at least, you're contributing to making the world a slightly less toxic place.

In the next few chapters, you'll learn exactly how to make 34 homemade shampoos. For your convenience the recipes have been grouped into chapters depending on the hair type they are best suited to. Check them out and enjoy!

Chapter 2

Insider Tips On Creating Your Own Shampoos

Creating your own shampoo can be quite an experience. Not only do you get to create something amazing for your hair, you also have the opportunity to learn more about how different ingredients can give your hair a healthy and natural shine without the need for chemical products.

It doesn't matter where you got your inspiration from, the important thing is that you've taken that first step to a much healthier, natural shampooing habit. Making your own shampoos will be a lot of fun, but there are some things you should be aware of before you begin. So before you grab that mixing bowl, here are a few insider tips to get you off to a good start and help you avoid any problems further down the road.

Prep your workspace

The first thing you need to do before you get started on your shampoo creations is to prep your workspace. Making your own shampoo at home can get quite messy, so make sure that you have prepared a dedicated space for it which will be easy to clean up when you've finished. Working in the kitchen is perfectly fine, but if you're going to turn it into a habit, you might want to look around your home for a small area you can dedicate to shampoo creation, space permitting of course.

Source your ingredients from a reliable supplier

Most of the ingredients needed to make your own homemade shampoo can easily be bought from grocery stores. However, if you're looking for an ingredient that can't be easily purchased in your area, you can always find a reliable supplier online with a little searching. When sourcing ingredients, make sure to choose a supplier that is known first and foremost for their quality, and not just the quantity of product they are offering. Don't be fooled by a cheap price tag if you're not sure about the quality of the product. Think of these ingredients as you would food; they will be entering your body through your scalp, so chose the best you can find or that you can afford.

Be aware of your allergies

Just because an ingredient is considered all-natural or organic doesn't mean that it's guaranteed to be 100% safe for you. It may work wonders for others, but there is the odd chance that for you it could cause an allergic reaction. So before you get started on any homemade shampoo batches, make sure that the ingredients you're going to use are safe for you. Try to figure out which (if any) of the common ingredients may cause skin irritation. If you're going to work with an unfamiliar ingredient, test it first on your wrist to see if it causes a negative reaction. This way, you don't end up harming your scalp or skin in your quest for healthier shampoo alternatives.

Start with small batches

Since your homemade shampoo doesn't contain any chemical ingredients designed to prolong its lifespan, it's best to only make small batches at a time. Most of the recipes for the DIY shampoo in this book will last for a matter of days or weeks, depending on the product. Therefore, it's highly recommended that you don't make too much at one time. One option to make your homemade shampoos last longer is to store them in the fridge. However, as making fresh batches is quick, easy and fun, creating more is unlikely to be a major inconvenience!

Always store homemade shampoo in appropriate containers

Once you've made a fresh batch of DIY shampoo, it's critical that you store it in an appropriate container. As I mentioned above, your homemade shampoo won't contain any chemical preservatives to prevent bacterial growth, so always make it a point to use sterile containers. Look for containers with airtight lids so your product won't be exposed to air, humidity, germs, and bacteria. Although not essential, glass containers are a good option as glass is inert, meaning no chemicals will be able to leach into your shampoos.

Don't get too hung up on following the recipes to the letter

The amounts of the ingredients you'll need may sometimes seem a little vague, but don't get too hung up on being exact; just follow the instructions as best you can to begin with. Making your own shampoos is a lot like cooking; over time you'll get used to the recipes and will be able to adjust them to suit your own needs and preferences.

Now that you're well prepared, let's get started on the recipes! Ive broken the recipes down into chapters based on type so if you like you can go straight to the chapter that interests you most. Good luck!

Chapter 3

The Quickest, Easiest Homemade Shampoo of Them All!

If you're feeling a little apprehensive about making your first homemade shampoo, fear not! There's one unbelievably simple but super-effective shampoo recipe. It may not contain the nourishing and fragrant ingredients of some of the other shampoos I share with you later in this book, but it is a great place to get started.

So what is this shampoo?

Well, the most basic homemade shampoo is made by simply mixing together baking soda and water. This shampoo is great as it clarifies the hair without stripping too much of the natural oil. Other benefits of using this shampoo include:

1. **Your hair will look more lively and vibrant.** Dry, limp hair is not only difficult to style, it can leave us feeling less than happy with the way we look. Using this simple baking soda and water recipe as an alternative to regular shampoo will help remedy this situation.

2. **It cleans without leaving a residue.** One problem with a lot of store-bought shampoos is

that they often leave behind a residue in the hair after washing. Due to the harsh nature of many of the ingredients used in these shampoos, this residue can cause the scalp to feel itchy and sensitive.

3. **It helps stop scalp irritation.** Baking soda will help defend your scalp from irritants and allergens. This can help prevent redness and flakiness — especially useful for those who's scalp is already sensitive.

4. **You probably already have the ingredients at home!** Not only will this simple shampoo alternative be better for your

hair, baking soda is inexpensive, and easy to get hold of.

Now you've been introduced to some of the benefits of this super-simple shampoo alternative, let's get to the recipe!

1. Easy-Peasy Homemade Shampoo

Ingredients:

- 3 cups water

- 1 cup baking soda

Instructions:

1. Mix the 3 cups of water with the 1 cup of baking soda in a large bowl. Be sure to wash this bowl well after use as you don't want to ingest any residue the baking soda may leave behind.

2. Make sure the mixture isn't clumpy and that the water and baking soda are mixed together thoroughly.

3. To apply, put a generous amount on your palms and massage it into your hair. An alternative method of application is to pour the mixture into a spray bottle and apply by spraying onto your hair.

4. Rinse as you would with a regular shampoo. Alternatively, for extra shine, use apple cider vinegar to rinse before a final rinse using cool water.

Congratulations! You've made your first natural Shampoo! See? That wasn't so hard, was it? OK, so we didn't include any fragrant, nourishing ingredients in this recipe, but we did make a simple alternative to store-bought shampoo.

If you're keen for more of a challenge, the next few chapters contain many more recipes, each of which require numerous ingredients to create. Don't be put off though as none of the recipes are difficult and if you follow the simple step by step instructions you'll be creating amazing shampoos in no time!

For your convenience, I've ordered the recipes in the next chapter so the the ones which require easy to find ingredients are listed first. There are a few recipes which require ingredients that might be a little harder to source (Google is a great place to look if you can't find the ingredients locally!), but they have been listed later in the chapter with a handy note beforehand. Good luck, and most of all, have fun!

Chapter 4

Homemade Shampoos for All Hair Types

Whatever type of hair you have, you can be sure that there are homemade shampoos that will be perfect for you. In this chapter you'll learn how to make shampoos that are suitable for all hair types. However, if you're having trouble with particularly dry hair and the shampoos in this chapter don't provide the required nourishment, I've included a chapter especially for you a little later on! If your hair is dry, simply skip ahead to chapter five, then when your hair recovers, come back to this chapter and give any recipes you like the sound of a try.

Similarly, if your hair is greasy or overly oily, I recommend you start by trying the recipes in chapter six. These recipes include ingredients which will strip away excess oil and grease without over-stimulating your scalp and hair follicles, meaning that your hair should regain its natural balance after just a few washes.

One more point before we start; I've created these recipes as I believe the ingredients combine well together and give shampoos which both smell great and leave hair feeling fantastic. However, after you have some experience, don't be afraid to experiment and adjust the recipes, adding and subtracting ingredients to suit your own particular tastes. Making homemade shampoos is a lot like cooking; experiment and tweak the recipes to suit your preferences.

For now, let's get started with Calming Chamomile and Rosemary Shampoo.

2. Calming Chamomile and Rosemary Shampoo

Everyone knows chamomile tea is refreshing and calming. A lesser known fact is that chamomile is also makes a fantastic homemade shampoo ingredient!

Ingredients:

- 2 cups of water infused with chamomile flowers (a couple of good quality chamomile tea bags will suffice if you really can't get the flowers), a palm full of rose petals, and a sprig or two of rosemary

- 5 drops rosemary essential oil

- 10 drops tea tree oil

- 15 drops chamomile essential oil

- ½ cup mild liquid castile soap

Instructions:

1. Pour the herb-infused water into a bowl.

2. Add the chamomile oil, rosemary oil, tea tree oil, and castile soap.

3. Mix until well-combined.

4. Use as you would a regular shampoo and rinse well with fresh cool water after use.

3. Peppermint and Rosemary Shampoo

This shampoo has a minty, fresh fragrance that leaves the scalp feeling cool and the hair looking and feeling wonderfully smooth!

Ingredients:

- 15 drops rosemary essential oil

- 2 drops peppermint essential oil

- ½ cup filtered water

- ½ cup mild liquid castile soap

Instructions:

1. Pour the liquid castile soap into a bottle.

2. Add the filtered water followed by the peppermint and rosemary essential oils.

3. Close the bottle and shake until the ingredients have been mixed well.

4. Use the way you would a regular shampoo and don't forget to give your hair and scalp a good rinse with fresh cool water.

4. Lavender and Bergamot Milky Mix

Aside from smelling like heaven, the pH balancing nature of this shampoo makes it perfect for those with slightly oily hair. The lavender in this shampoo can also help promote a restful night's sleep.

Ingredients:

- 8 drops of lavender essential oil

- 6 drops of bergamot oil

- ½ cup mild liquid castile soap

- ¼ cup coconut milk

Instructions:

1. Pour the liquid castile soap in a bottle followed by the coconut milk.

2. Add the bergamot and lavender oil and shake well until the ingredients are thoroughly combined.

3. Use the way you would a regular shampoo then rinse with cool water after use.

5. Avocado Aloe Surprise

Use this shampoo before a long day in the sun, to prevent it from drying out or becoming heat-damaged so you can spend less time worrying about the condition of your hair and more on enjoying the lovely weather!

Ingredients:

- ¼ tsp organic avocado oil

- 1 tsp 100% pure glycerin

- ¼ cup aloe vera gel

- ¼ cup pure liquid castile soap

Instructions:

1. Pour the liquid castile soap into a bowl.

2. Add the glycerin, avocado oil, and aloe vera gel.

3. Stir until well-combined then transfer the mixture to a suitable container.

4. Before using this shampoo, make sure that you first shake well.

5. Massage onto your hair and leave for 5 to 10 minutes before rinsing with cool water.

6. A Little Bit of Sunshine

With the inclusion of lemon zest and orange essential oil, this shampoo is so fantastic that no matter how limp and tired you think your hair looks, "A little Bit of Sunshine" is sure to bring back it's luster! Oh, and it smells great too!

Ingredients:

- ¼ cup water

- 5 drops orange essential oil

- 6 drops chamomile essential oil

- 3 drops rose essential oil

- 1 tsp fresh lemon zest

- ¼ cup pure liquid castile soap

Instructions:

1. Pour the liquid castile soap in a microwave-safe bowl.

2. Add the lemon zest, rose essential oil, chamomile essential oil, and orange essential oil.

3. Add the water and mix until well combined.

4. Place the bowl in the microwave and heat for around two minutes. Adjust this time as necessary; we want the mixture to be hot but not boiling.

5. Let the mixture cool then transfer it to a bottle and keep in a cool, dry place.

6. Use this shampoo as you would a regular store-bought shampoo, and after use, rinse with cool water.

7. Surprisingly Good Apple & Garlic Shampoo

Even though garlic is used as one of the ingredients, this shampoo actually smells great! Don't be put off by the garlic; give this shampoo a try and judge for yourself. Especially useful for those who suffer from dandruff.

Ingredients:

- ½ cup grape seed oil

- ¼ cup liquid castile soap

- ¼ cup water

- 6 finely crushed garlic cloves

- 3 tbsp fresh apple juice

- 1 tbsp apple cider vinegar

Instructions:

1. Pour the liquid castile soap into a food processor.

2. Add the grape seed oil, garlic cloves, apple cider vinegar, apple juice, and distilled water.

3. Pulse until smooth and similar to the the consistency of a regular store-bought shampoo.

4. Don't forget to rinse with cool water after you've washed. If you're worried that others may be able to smell the garlic, simply rinse your hair with apple cider vinegar or lemon juice before rinsing with cool water.

8. Shining Shimmering Splendid Shampoo

As well as leaving your hair looking silky-smooth, the mixture of essential oils included in the recipe give this shampoo a refreshing and calming effect.

Ingredients:

- ¼ cup boiled distilled water

- ½ tsp lemon essential oil

- 2 Tbsp almond oil

- ½ tsp jasmine essential oil

- ½ tsp vanilla essential oil

- 2 tbsp dried rosemary (not powdered rosemary!)

- ¼ cup liquid castile soap

Instructions:

1. Pour the boiled water over the dried rosemary to make an infusion.

2. Let the infusion cool by steeping it for two or three minutes.

3. Once the infusion has cooled, strain it. This liquid will form the base of the shampoo.

4. Add the vanilla, lemon, and jasmine essential oils, followed by the almond oil and the liquid castile soap.

5. Stir until well combined. If you prefer you can pour the mixture into a suitable container then shake until the ingredients are well mixed.

6. Use the way you would a regular shampoo and don't forget to rinse with cool water.

9. Lovely Lemony Egg Shampoo

The beauty of using egg in your homemade hair products is that it's a fantastic natural moisturizer which leaves your hair super-smooth and looking great! Follow these simple steps to make this wonderful shampoo.

Ingredients:

- 3 tsp baking soda

- 2 eggs

- 2 tsp lemon juice

- 2 tsp olive oil

Instructions:

1. Beat the eggs in a bowl until well mixed.

2. Next, add the olive oil, lemon juice, and baking soda and mix.

3. Pour the mixture into a suitable container. Shake well before use.

4. Apply to your hair by massaging it from your scalp to the tips.

5. Rinse well with cool water.

10. Miraculous Apple Cider Shampoo

Apple cider vinegar is great for helping to make hair silky smooth. As a bonus, it also helps in promoting hair growth!

Ingredients:

- 30 ml olive oil

- 3 drops eucalyptus essential oil

- 1 tsp apple cider vinegar

- 2 tsp fresh lemon juice

- 1 egg

Instructions:

1. Put the lemon juice, apple cider vinegar, eucalyptus oil, olive oil, and egg into a food processor.

2. Pulse until smooth.

3. Transfer contents to a suitable container.

4. To use this shampoo, simply massage into your hair and leave it on for at least 5 minutes before rinsing with cool water.

11. Awesome Aromatherapy Shampoo

Jojoba Oil is not only super-nourishing, it also smells great and helps give the hair volume. Meanwhile, the Ylang-Ylang oil in this recipe is naturally calming, making this shampoo perfect for hydrating the hair while at the same time helping you feel rejuvenated and happy!

Ingredients:

- 5 drops ylang-ylang oil

- 10 drops rosemary oil

- 40 drops lavender oil

- 1 Tbsp jojoba oil

- ¼ cup pure liquid castile soap

Instructions:

1. Pour the liquid castile soap into a bowl.

2. Add the jojoba, lavender, rosemary, and ylang-ylang oils.

3. Mix well.

4. Transfer the mixture to a bottle and shake.

5. Shampoo your hair the way you would normally, then rinse with cool water.

12. Chamomile and Apricot Shampoo

Apricot is often used in products to help nourish the skin. Well, you'll be glad to know that you can also use apricot to treat your hair and scalp! This shampoo is great if you have kids, as the chamomile is especially gentle on sensitive skin.

Ingredients:

- 1 tsp apricot oil

- ¼ cup fresh rosemary herbs

- 1/8 tsp dried dandelion leaves

- 1 cup distilled water

- 2 drops chamomile essential oil

Instructions:

1. Place the dandelion leaves, rosemary herbs, chamomile oil and apricot oil in a food processor.

2. Pour in the distilled water.

3. Process until smooth then transfer the contents to a suitable container.

4. Apply as you would a regular shampoo and use cool water to rinse.

13. Shiny Strawberry Shampoo

The amazing scent of strawberries is loved by people around the world, and the strawberry in this recipe will leave your hair smelling great! In addition, the tea tree oil is great at cleaning away dirt and excess oil.

Ingredients:

- 1 cup strawberries, crushed

- 3 tsp xanthan gum

- ¼ cup pure liquid castile soap

- ¼ cup baking soda

- 3 drops tea tree oil

- 2 cups distilled water

Instructions:

1. Put the crushed strawberries into a food processor and pulse until smooth.

2. Pour the distilled water into a pot and add the strawberry paste.

3. Add the xanthan gum, castile soap, tea tree oil and baking soda.

4. Heat gently on the stove until everything has been thoroughly mixed and the desired consistency has been achieved.

5. Let the mixture cool for a while then transfer to a suitable container.

6. Shake the container well before use.

7. Massage into your hair and scalp as you would a regular shampoo.

8. Don't forget to rinse with cool water afterwards!

14. Anti-Damage Shampoo

This shampoo is fantastic for bringing dull and damaged hair back to life, giving it a smooth and soft appearance while at the same time offering protection against future damage.

Ingredients:

- 5 drops lemon essential oil

- ½ cup distilled water

- 1 tsp lemon juice

- 1 tsp coconut oil

- 1 large egg

- 1 tsp organic coconut oil

Instructions:

1. Place the large egg in a blender, followed by coconut oil, lemon juice, essential oil and distilled water.

2. Process until smooth and well blended then transfer the mixture to a suitable container.

3. To use, simply massage into your hair and leave for a couple of minutes before rinsing with cool water.

15. Merry Minty Rosemary

The mint leaves and peppermint oil used in this shampoo recipe are perfect for helping to keep your hair and scalp feeling cool and clean during the summer months!

Ingredients:

- 1 drop rosemary essential oil

- 2 tbsp mint leaves

- 1 cup boiled water

- 2 drops peppermint essential oil

- 2 tbsp castile oil

Instructions:

1. Put the mint leaves in a cup or small bowl and pour in the boiled water. Make sure all the mint leaves are fully immersed in the water.

2. Let steep for 15 to 20 minutes. Gently agitate the leaves once or twice during this time.

3. Strain and keep the liquid. Discard the mint leaves.

4. Let cool at room temperature before adding the peppermint oil, rosemary oils and the castile oil.

5. Transfer the contents to a suitable container.

6. To use, simply massage into your hair and leave for a couple of minutes before rinsing with cool water.

16. Ring around the Rosy

The scent of rose is simply wonderful and is known to evoke feelings of romance and warmth.

Ingredients:

- 3 drops essential rose oil

- 3 tbsp castile soap, grated

- 1 tbsp organic coconut oil

- ¼ cup organic coconut milk

- ¼ cup organic rose petals

- ½ cup hot water

Instructions:

1. Put the rose petals in the hot water and leave for at least 30 minutes.

2. Use a strainer to strain the liquid. Discard the petals and use the liquid. Let it cool before adding the rest of the ingredients.

3. Add the coconut milk, coconut oil, castile soap, and rose oil and mix by whisking.

4. Transfer the contents to a bottle and use the way you would a regular shampoo.

5. Rinse well with cool water.

17. The Fine Pine

The pine oil in this recipe acts as a fantastic natural moisturizer, while the cypress, lemongrass and tea tree oils clean your hair and leave it smelling great!

Ingredients:

- 15 drops pine essential oil

- 4 drops cypress essential oil

- 10 drops lemongrass essential oil

- ½ tsp tea tree essential oil

- 1/3 cup decyl glucoside (If you can't get this, an alternative is to simply replace with 3 tbsps castile soap in 1/3 cup of warm water.)

- 1/3 cup raw honey

- 1/3 cup water

Instructions:

1. Put the pine, cypress, and lemongrass essential oils into a bowl.

2. Add the tea tree oil and decyl glucoside along with the honey.

3. Pour on the water and stir until well mixed.

4. Transfer into a suitable container and use as needed.

5. To use, simply massage the mixture into your hair and scalp as you would a regular shampoo.

6. Rinse with cool water.

18. Aloe, Nettle, and Papaya Shampoo

As well as being a great all-round shampoo, *this recipe is great if you're suffering from thinning or brittle hair.*

Ingredients:

- A handful of nettle (be careful!)

- 1 cup hot water

- 1 tbsp aloe vera

- 1 large papaya

Instructions:

1. Infuse the hot water with the nettle. Leave for at least 30 minutes and then strain. Discard nettle and leave the liquid to cool.

2. Place the papaya and aloe vera in a food processor.

3. Pulse until a smooth shampoo-like consistency is achieved.

4. Add the nettle-infused water and pulse until well mixed.

5. Leave until cool and then transfer to a suitable container.

6. Use as you would a regular shampoo.

7. Rinse with cool water.

Note: The ingredients for the next few shampoos may be a little harder to get hold of, but if you shop around online you can usually find them fairly easily and at a reasonable price. Despite the fact that you might have to hunt around a little for the ingredients, these shampoos are well worth giving a try if you've enjoyed making some of the previous shampoos and are ready for a bit more of a challenge!

19. Fantastic Fenugreek Shampoo

You know what's great about Fenugreek? It naturally encourages hair growth because it is full of protein, lecithin, and amino acids. These ingredients also help keep your hair strong and your scalp in good condition

Ingredients:

- A bowl of water

- 2 tbsp Fenugreek seeds

Instructions:

1. In 1 to 2 cups of water, soak the unprocessed fenugreek seeds overnight.

2. Prepare the seeds by straining the water and placing them in a food processor.

3. Pulse until a smooth and finely ground consistency is achieved.

4. Apply this mixture to your scalp using your fingers then let it stay there for around 40 minutes.

5. Rinse with a mix of water, lemon and vinegar, or simply by using cool water alone.

20. Sandalwood and Chamomile Surprise

While the smell of sandalwood may be a little too strong for some, it combines fantastically with chamomile. This shampoo helps to strengthen hair, making this recipe especially good for those with thinner hair.

Ingredients:

- 25 grams dried soapwort root

- 20 drops sandalwood oil

- 25 grams dry chamomile flowers

- 1 cup hot water

Instructions:

1. Prepare a bowl of hot water and place the soapwort root and chamomile flowers inside. Make sure the soapwort root and chamomile flowers are fully immersed in the water.

2. Leave the mixture overnight (or for at least 12 hours).

3. Add the sandalwood oil and stir until the ingredients have been mixed thoroughly.

4. Transfer to a suitable container and use the way you would a regular shampoo.

5. Rinse well with cool water after use.

21. Dandruff-Busting Neem Leaf Shampoo

As the name suggests, this shampoo is fantastic for combatting dandruff. It also contains anti-fungal properties that will help prevent your scalp from flaking or itching.

Ingredients:

- 4 to 5 cups hot water

- 2 handfuls of neem leaves

Instructions:

1. Put the neem leaves in a bowl filled with hot water and allow to sit overnight (or for at least 8 hours).

2. Use a strainer to strain the liquid then pour this liquid into a suitable container.

3. Massage this into your scalp and hair and leave for at least an hour. To prevent the liquid evaporating I recommend wrapping your head in a warm, damp towel.

4. Rinse with cool water, dry, and style your hair. For best results allow your hair to dry naturally, or at the very least, avoid using the higher heat settings on your hairdryer.

22. Amazing Ayurvedic Shampoo

The ingredients used in this shampoo are very popular Ayurvedic elements, so when you use this shampoo you're not only nourishing your hair, you're also nourishing your soul! Believe it or not, this shampoo can also be used as a face or body wash, making it all the more incredible!

Ingredients:

- 1 to 2 tsp shikakai powder

- 100 grams soap nuts

Instructions:

1. Put the soap nuts in a bowl and add enough water to cover them. Soak overnight (or for at least 8 hours).

2. The following day, remove the water and pour the soaked soap nuts into a blender.

3. Add the shikakai powder.

4. Process until the mixture has a smooth consistency.

5. To use, massage the mixture onto your hair. Leave for at least 15 minutes before rinsing with cool water. You can also rinse the hair with lemon infused water for extra shine, if desired.

23. Curry for the Hair

This is another Ayurveda-inspired shampoo recipe. While many think curry leaves are simply of use for adding flavor to food, you may be surprised to learn that they can also do wonders for your hair!

Ingredients:

- 250 grams fenugreek

- 500 grams shikakai

- 100 grams soap beans

- A bunch of basil leaves

- A bunch of curry leaves

- 250 grams mung beans

Instructions:

1. Lay down the fenugreek, shikakai, basil leaves, soap beans, curry leaves, and mung beans on paper and leave them to sun-dry for at least 12 hours.

2. When these ingredients have dried out, place them all in a food processor and process until smooth.

3. Store the paste in a suitable container.

4. To use, mix a small amount with water and massage into your hair.

5. Rinse well with cool water being careful to check that no residue is left behind.

24. Black Soap Shampoo

African black soap is a mixture of Shea butter, palm kernel oil, plantain and cocoa pod ash. It's not only great for the skin but also for the hair, and can help with a dry scalp, dandruff, and tangled, frizzy hair!

Ingredients:

- 3 tbsp grape seed oil

- 2 tbsp raw honey

- 1 cup hot water

- 4 tbsp African black soap, crumbled

Instructions:

1. Put the African soap, raw honey, and grape seed oil into a suitable container.

2. Pour the hot water over the ingredients.

3. Fasten the container securely and shake until all of the ingredients have been thoroughly mixed.

4. Lather on your hair gently then rinse well with warm or cool water.

Chapter 5

Homemade Shampoos for Dry Hair

Your hair can become overly-dry for a number of reasons. Common causes of this frustrating condition are the weather and our lifestyle choices. However, if you suffer from dry hair it's possible that the reason may be a little less obvious; certain ingredients in store bought shampoos can trigger allergies without you even being aware of the fact. If you're not sure whether or not your hair should be classified as "dry", look out for these telltale signs:

1. **Your hair looks and feels limp**. This is often an indication that we've used too many styling products, which introduce harmful chemicals to our hair and scalp. It can also indicate that our hair has been damaged by the heat from our hairdryers, hair irons or curlers. This in turn can cause the hair to look limp and frizzy.

2. **You have many split ends.** No matter how beautiful the majority of our hair is, split ends can really detract from it's overall appearance. Again, split ends are usually caused by excess heat.

3. **Your hair is usually dull and lacks a healthy shine**. This tends to indicate that the hair has been damaged by harsh chemicals in commercial styling products. These chemicals can strip the hair of it's natural oils. When the oil has been removed the hair is more susceptible to damage, which in turn causes it to appear dull.

4. **Your hair easily sheds or breaks**. If you're finding yourself losing an unusual amount of hair in a short period of time this is an indication that you may be suffering from dry hair. Times when you may typically notice your hair breaking are when brushing, styling or tying.

5. **Your hair tangles easily**. If your hair tangles easily and is difficult to separate without breaking, you may well be suffering from dry hair. Again, this occurs due to the stripping of the hair's natural oils. When this happens the strands of hair are unable to "slide" over one another smoothly leading to tangles, and in more severe cases, knots.

If you're experiencing any of these symptoms then chances are you're suffering from dry hair. But don't worry, because on the next few pages you'll learn how to make some excellent homemade shampoos for dry hair. Turn to the next page to get started!

25. More Honey, No Problems

Honey is a great ingredient as it has anti-fungal and anti-bacterial properties. Try this soothing shampoo recipe and your dry hair should begin to clear up in no time!

Ingredients:

- 3 tbsp water (filtered is best)

- 1 tbsp raw or unpasteurized honey (regular honey will do in a pinch, but the aforementioned types are definitely preferable!)

- 5 to 10 drops of carrot seed oil

Instructions:

1. Mix the 3 tablespoons of water with the 1 tablespoon of raw honey.

2. Gently heat the mixture so that honey dissolves. Fully dissolve the honey being sure to keep the heat low.

3. Add 5 to 10 drops of carrot seed oil. This can help prevent your hair from flaking and your scalp from itching.

4. To use, simply wet your hair and massage the shampoo into your hair and scalp.

5. Rinse well with cool water.

26. Coconut Milk Shampoo

The combination of Coconut Milk, Olive Oil, and Castile Soap in this recipe is guaranteed to leave your hair feeling smooth and moisturized. What's more, it's super quick and easy to make!

Ingredients:

- 3 tbsps organic coconut milk

- ¼ cup liquid castile soap

- 1 tsp olive oil

- 1 tsp distilled water

Instructions:

1. Pour the coconut milk, castile soap, water and olive oil into a small container.

2. Shake the container well until the ingredients are mixed thoroughly.

3. Use the way you would a regular shampoo and rinse with cool water or apple cider vinegar.

27. Cool Cucumber and Lemon Shampoo

This cucumber and lemon shampoo is so soothing you'll forget that you ever had dry hair. It also smells wonderful!

Ingredients:

- 1 whole cucumber

- 1 whole lemon

Instructions:

1. Place the cucumber and lemon in your food processor. (You don't need to worry about

peeling the lemon, but if you'd prefer a smoother shampoo you can if you like.)

2. Pulse until you get a mixture that has a shampoo-like consistency.

3. Put a generous amount on your palms and rub into your hair and scalp.

4. Rinse well with cool water.

Chapter 6

Homemade Shampoos for Greasy & Oily Hair

In this chapter we have some homemade shampoo recipes that are perfect for oily and greasy hair. Usually, oily hair is caused by either using too much shampoo or using a shampoo that's too harsh for your scalp. However, other causes can be eating an unbalanced diet or eating food products that you are allergic to. In addition, excess oil production from the scalp can be caused by stress and can even occur due to certain weather conditions.

Whatever the cause, oily hair can make styling a real chore! Not only that, but as anyone who has suffered from this condition will be able to tell you, having oily hair can be a massive confidence drain. Greasy hair oftentimes has a "dirty" look to it which can cause major embarrassment and leave you feeling far less than your best.

If you're suffering from oily, greasy hair, make sure that you give these natural shampoos a try!

28. Green-Goodness Shampoo

This shampoo is super gentle, making it great for those who have a sensitive scalp and oily hair. It also lathers well, meaning you'll really be able to coat your hair thoroughly to get rid of that icky grease!

Ingredients:

- 10 drops tea tree oil

- 2 tsp green tea, brewed strongly (drink the rest; it's fantastic for your health!)

- 1 tbsp liquid castile soap

- 1 tbsp green clay

Instructions:

1. Mix the castile soap, green clay, green tea, and tea tree oil together in a bowl.

2. Stir until the mixture turns a muddy green color.

3. Massage well into your hair and scalp until bubbly.

4. Rinse well with cool water.

29. Avocado and Castile Shampoo

Another wonderful homemade shampoo for those whose hair tends to be greasy. This simple shampoo will help rebalance the production of natural oils from the scalp.

Ingredients:

- ¼ cup avocado oil

- 120 grams castile flakes

- ¼ gallon water

Instructions:

1. Boil the water.

2. Put the flakes in a large, heat-proof bowl.

3. When boiled, pour the water over the flakes.

4. Stir mixture until cool then add the avocado oil.

5. Pour the mixture into a suitable container then use as you would a regular shampoo.

6. Rinse with cool water.

30. All Hail Lemon and Aloe

Aloe Vera is one of the best natural products when it comes to aiding healthy hair growth and preventing hair from becoming excessively oily. This shampoo also smells fantastic, leaving you feeling refreshed and relaxed after use!

Ingredients:

- 2 tbsp lemon juice, freshly squeezed

- 1 tsp aloe vera gel

- ½ cup liquid castile soap

Instructions:

1. Pour the liquid castile soap into a suitable container.

2. Add the aloe vera gel and the freshly squeezed lemon juice.

3. Shake container well until the ingredients are mixed well.

4. Use as you would a regular shampoo and rinse with cool water after.

Chapter 7

Homemade Dry Shampoos

Finally, in this chapter I'll be showing you how to make homemade dry shampoos. When using these shampoos there's no need to rinse, making them super quick and easy alternatives to regular shampoos. Some of the other benefits of using dry shampoos include:

1. **They make your hair softer**. Natural dry shampoos give the hair a healthy shine and make it extremely soft.

2. **They can save you a lot of time**. As mentioned above, when using a dry shampoo you won't have to rinse your hair, and this in turn means you won't have to worry about drying it either. This can obviously help you save a lot of time which can be especially beneficial if you're the type of person who's always on the go.

3. **They give your hair volume.** Hair with volume looks beautiful and healthy, and one way to achieve healthy volume is to use dry shampoos. They can help your hair retain more of it's natural volume as you're not constantly wetting it down and then drying it out.

4. **If your hair has been colored, dry shampoos can help to maintain the color longer.** The harsh chemicals in commercially available liquid shampoos can strip the color from colored hair; not what you want if you've recently been to the salon for an expensive color treatment!

5. **The hair's natural oils remain intact.** This again is due to the fact that when using natural homemade shampoos you're not exposing your hair to the harsh chemicals in store bought shampoos, nor are you regularly rinsing the hair with water. This helps the hair to retain it's natural oils which in turn will keep it looking naturally healthy!

6. **No need for drying means less heat damage!** As you don't need to wet your hair when using dry shampoos, you also don't need to dry it with a hairdryer. No drying equals less heat damage!

Turn over to the next page to learn how to make a selection of dry shampoos. If you've never used them before, why not try them out; you might be pleasantly surprised by the results!

31. Lavender and Arrowroot Shampoo

The lavender in this dry shampoo can help promote a restful night's sleep, so its a great dry shampoo to use if you're cleaning your hair before going to bed. Arrowroot, meanwhile, is full of proteins that can strengthen the hair via the scalp.

Ingredients:

- 5 drops lavender essential oil

- ¼ cup arrowroot powder

Instructions:

1. Put the arrowroot powder into a small bowl.

2. Add the lavender essential oil and use a spoon to mix together thoroughly.

3. Store the dry shampoo in an old powder container or a mason jar. (Make sure the container is sealed tightly so no moisture can enter.)

4. Apply the dry shampoo with your hands, being sure to gently rub it into both your hair and your scalp.

5. There's no need to rinse; simply comb the shampoo out of your hair (I recommend doing this over the sink to minimize any mess!) and style as usual.

32. Dry Cornmeal and Salt Shampoo

This shampoo is great for removing dirt and oil from your hair and it also helps keep the hair silky smooth. Give this super quick and easy shampoo a go next time you're in a rush!

Ingredients:

- ½ cup cornmeal

- 1 tbsp sea salt or pink Himalayan salt (finely ground)

Instructions:

1. Put the cornmeal and the salt in a bowl together.

2. Mix until well-combined then transfer to a pepper shaker or an old powder container.

3. Apply the dry shampoo with your hands, being sure to gently rub it into both your hair and your scalp.

4. There's no need to rinse; simply comb the shampoo out of your hair (I recommend doing this over the sink to minimize any mess!) and style as usual.

33. Almond and Orris Root Shampoo

This gentle shampoo will keep your hair looking healthy and feeling smooth. It also smells absolutely fantastic!

Ingredients:

- 1 tbsp orris root

- 1 tbsp cornmeal

- 1 tbsp finely ground almonds

Instructions:

1. In a bowl, mix together the cornmeal, orris root, and almonds.

2. Transfer to a pepper shaker or an old powder container.

3. Apply the dry shampoo with your hands, being sure to gently rub it into both your hair and your scalp.

4. There's no need to rinse; simply comb the shampoo out of your hair (I recommend doing this over the sink to minimize any mess!) and style as usual.

34. Dry Baking Soda and Oatmeal Shampoo

Many people know of Oatmeal's use in making natural skin exfoliators, but not so many know that it can also be used to smoothen and strengthen the hair. Try this recipe to see just how effective it can be.

Ingredients:

- 1 cup baking soda

- 1 cup oatmeal

Instructions:

1. In a bowl, mix the oatmeal and the baking soda together.

2. Mix well until the ingredients are combined.

3. Transfer the mixture to a bottle or old powder container.

4. Apply the dry shampoo with your hands, being sure to gently rub it in to both your hair and your scalp.

5. As with the other dry shampoos, there's no need to rinse; simply comb the shampoo out of your hair (I recommend doing this over the sink to minimize any mess!) and style as usual.

Conclusion

The way we choose to spend our money is important. If we continue to support companies that make a profit from endangering our health, it could be said that we are exercising poor judgment and failing to act wisely.

I believe it's important that we each do our own research into the shampoos we buy and use. For our health's sake, as well as the health of others who use these products, it pays to be an informed consumer and to vote with our dollars.

Thank you again for downloading this book. I hope you enjoyed reading it and were able to learn a lot about the benefits of making your own shampoo at home. What's more, I hope you will actually try some of the recipes for yourself and that you're able to experience the benefits of using these natural, healthy alternatives to store-bought shampoos.

A message from the author, Jane Aniston

Finally, if you enjoyed this book, **please** take the time to post a review on Amazon. It will only take a couple of minutes and I'd be extremely grateful for your support. Thank you.

Jane Aniston

FREE BONUS!: Preview Of

"Homemade Makeup - A

Complete Beginner's Guide to

Natural DIY Cosmetics You Can

Make Today" - Includes 28 Organic

Makeup Recipes!'

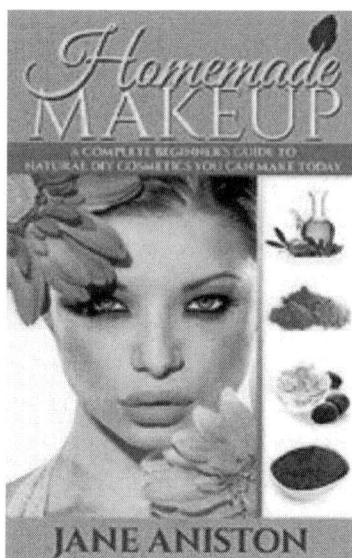

If you enjoyed this book, I have a little bonus for you; a preview of one of my other books "Homemade Makeup - A Complete Beginner's Guide to Natural DIY Cosmetics You Can Make Today", which exposes the secrets of the hidden toxins lurking in your store-bought cosmetics! This book also includes 28 simple and enjoyable organic makeup recipes that you can make at home today. Give yourself a glamorous look without exposing yourself to potentially harmful chemical nasties! Enjoy!

Chapter 1: Why you should stop using store-bought makeup and start making your own at home!

Makeup is something most women simply can't live without. Some women, in their search for beauty, have even gone as far getting permanent cosmetics tattooed on their faces (permanent eyebrows, for example). Personally, I see nothing wrong with wanting to look your best, but at the end of the day, one question we need to ask ourselves is: "What exactly are the ingredients in my beauty products?"

With almost all cosmetics containing numerous chemical ingredients, it can be a bit unsettling to think about the potential long-term effects these ingredients could be having on our bodies. Behind the glamour of the cosmetics industry, there's always the danger that the products we think are safe to put on our skin, might in actuality not be as safe as we think.

After studying the cosmetics industry, the truth is that these products have some of the largest mark-ups of any you're likely to find on the high street or in the mall! Your favorite face cream that cost you $80 may well have only cost as little as $2 to make, while that trendy lipstick you paid $30 of your hard-earned money for may actually only have a monetary value of $0.75! If you've bought thousands of dollars worth of cosmetics over the years, this realization can be pretty depressing. It doesn't feel good to know that all this time we've been duped by the cosmetics industry via slick marketing campaigns, while they made massive profits out of us unsuspecting consumers.

This is certainly something I've been a victim of. In the past, one of the things I would regularly spend money on was a good (and very expensive!) lipstick. Whenever I was having a bad day, I would head down to my favorite store and treat myself to a new shade. My friends would easily be able to tell if I was having a good year or not by the number of lipsticks I had in my collection! In hindsight, knowing what I know now, I feel a real sense of regret that I didn't get around to making my own cosmetics earlier. If I had of done, my bank balance certainly would have been a little healthier, and that money could have been better put to use.

The thing about the cosmetics industry is that even if you have a suspicion you're being ripped-off, it just feels that buying these products is something you *have to do*. I know a lot of women who would gladly fork over an inordinate amount of money for an excellent foundation! Why? Because you simply can't put a price on the confidence that looking your best can give you. The marketing used to sell cosmetic products has preyed on the insecurities of women for far too long. We are constantly bombarded with the message that if you want to feel good about yourself you need to look like a cover model; the implication being that the only way you'll be able to do that is to use their (expensive!) cosmetics. It's even gotten to the point where some women consider certain brands of makeup to be status symbols, much like they may do with a pair of expensive shoes or a designer handbag.

Am I immune to the marketing hype surrounding cosmetics? Honestly, no. I confess that even after learning the heartbreaking truth about the beauty industry I still get excited when I'm in the store browsing the makeup department. I still look at each lipstick color and eye shadow shade and imagine how I would incorporate them to achieve all sorts of glamorous looks. The only difference now is I don't purchase anywhere near as many products as I used to. These days I usually just look around in search of color inspiration, make a mental note and then create my own cosmetics at home. If you're thinking that the only reason I do this is to save a few dollars, you're wrong. Unfortunately there's more to it than that.

Harmful Ingredients Abound!

One of the sad realities when it comes to cosmetics is that the vast majority contain toxic ingredients. Even makeup products labeled as "all-natural" often times contain ingredients that may increase susceptibility to skin allergies, cancer, infertility and reproductive problems. If you're not sure about which ingredients you'd be best to avoid, here's a list of chemical nasties which are often used in cosmetics. Considering that human skin absorbs almost 60% of what is applied to it, this list will make you think twice next time you're about to splurge on expensive cosmetics.

- **Coal Tar** – Although already banned in the EU and Southeast Asia, there are still some products being sold in the US that contain this carcinogen. It's often found in treatments for dry skin as well as in anti-dandruff shampoos. Coal tar is also known as FD&C Red No.6.

- **Ethoxylated surfactants and 1,4-dioxane** – Created when carcinogenic ethylene oxide is added to a cocktail of other chemicals. This nasty toxin is found in some cosmetics, and unfortunately, is commonly found in baby washes being sold in the US. As a general rule, if you want to err on the safe side, avoid ingredients that contain the syllable "eth".

- **Fragrance/"Parfum"** – A catchall for unknown chemicals like phthalates. Fragrance has been proven to cause dizziness, headaches, asthma, and even allergic reactions in some unsuspecting victims.

- **Formaldehyde** – A proven irritant and likely carcinogen that can be found in hair dye, nail products, and shampoos. It is already banned in the EU.

- **Lead** – A carcinogenic contaminant found in most lipsticks and hair dyes. Since it's not officially considered to be an ingredient, you'll never see this listed on any beauty product.

- **Hydroquinone** – An ingredient used to peal and lighten skin. It is banned in the UK due to the fact it's been linked to cancer and reproductive disorders.

- **Mineral oil** – This petroleum byproduct can be found in moisturizers, baby oils, and styling gels.

- **Mercury** – An allergen that is known to impair brain function and development. Can be found in select eye drops and mascaras.

- **Parabens** – Used to preserve ingredients in many beauty and baby products. Has been linked to cancer, reproductive disorders, and endocrine problems.

- **Oxybenzone** – A chemical sunscreen that accumulates in fat cells. It can cause allergic reactions and hormone irregularity.

- **Phthalates** – A type of plasticizer that is banned in the EU and just recently, in California. It can be found in perfumes, deodorants, and lotions; and has been linked to kidney, liver, and lung damage.

- **Paraphenylenediamine (PPD)** – Present in hair dyes and styling products. Proven to be toxic to skin and can cause complications with the immune system.

- **Silicone derived emollients** – An ingredient added to some cosmetic products to make them feel soft. It has been linked to skin irritation and tumor enlargement.

- **Talc** – Has a similar composition to asbestos. Can be found in some blushes, eye shadows, baby powders, and deodorants. Has been linked to respiratory problems and ovarian cancer.

- **Sodium lauryl (ether) sulphate (SLS, SLES)** – An ingredient added to soap to make it foamy. It's easily absorbed by the body and can lead to irritation of sensitive skin.

- **Triclosan** – Can be found in some hand sanitizers, deodorants, and antibacterial products. It has been linked to endocrine disorders and cancer.

- **Toluene** – Has been linked to endocrine and immune disorders. Often found in hair and nail products, this ingredient is often hidden under the term, "fragrance."

Check out the rest of "Homemade Makeup: A Complete Beginner's Guide To Natural DIY Cosmetics You Can Make Today" by Jane Aniston on Amazon.

Check Out My Other Books!

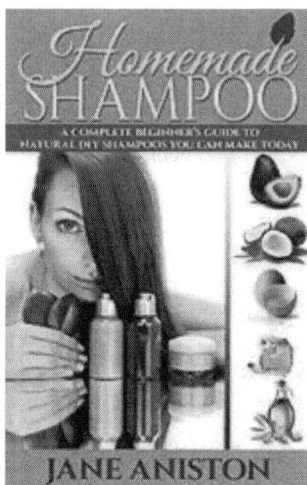

Homemade Shampoo (Includes 34 Organic Shampoo Recipes!)

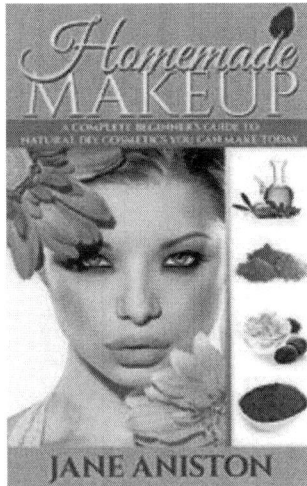

Homemade Makeup (Includes 28 Organic Makeup Recipes!)

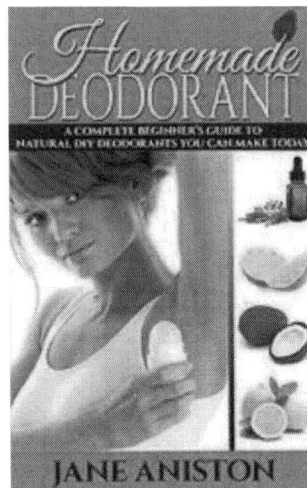

Homemade Deodorant (Includes 20 Organic Deodorant Recipes!)

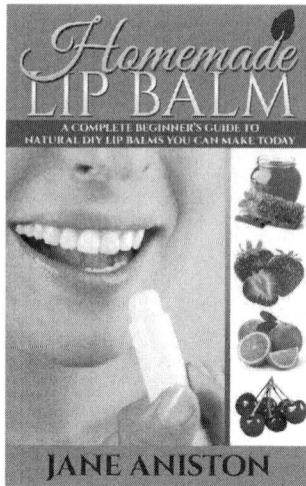

Homemade Lip Balm (Includes 22 Organic Lip Balm Recipes!)

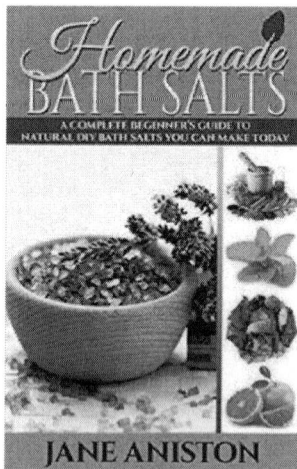

Homemade Bath Salts (Includes 35 Organic Bath Salt Recipes!)

Printed in Germany
by Amazon Distribution
GmbH, Leipzig